Paleo Slow Cooker Recipes

The Best Paleo Diet Recipes for Your Slow Cooker

Daisy Williams

This book is dedicated to those who value spending less time in the kitchen and still strive to prepare healthy meals for their families. With Paleo slow cooking; prep it, set and forget. You will soon find that slow cooking and the Paleo diet are two examples of the simpler things in life.

Copyright © 2014 by Speedy Publishing LLC

All rights reserved. No part of this publication may be reproduced, distributed or transmitted in any form or by any means, including photocopying, recording, or other electronic or mechanical methods, without the prior written permission of the publisher, except in the case of brief quotations embodied in critical reviews and certain other noncommercial uses permitted by copyright law. For permission requests, write to the publisher, addressed "Attention: Permissions Coordinator," at the address below.

Speedy Publishing LLC (c) 2014
40 E. Main St., #1156
Newark, DE 19711
www.speedypublishing.co

Ordering Information:
Quantity sales; Special discounts are available on quantity purchases by corporations, associations, and others. For details, contact the "Special Sales Department" at the address above.

-- 1st edition

Manufactured in the United States of America

Table of Contents

Publisher's Notes i

Chapter 1: What is Slow Cooking? 1

Chapter 2: What is the Paleo Diet? 5

Chapter 3: What are the Benefits of the Paleo Diet? 9

Chapter 4: 10 Slow Cooker Paleo Breakfast Recipes 13

Chapter 5: 10 Slow Cooker Paleo Lunch/Dinner Recipes 21

Chapter 6: 10 Slow Cooker Paleo Dessert Recipes 29

About the Author 38

More Books by Daisy Williams 40

PUBLISHER'S NOTES

Disclaimer

This publication is intended to provide helpful and informative material. It is not intended to diagnose, treat, cure, or prevent any health problem or condition, nor is intended to replace the advice of a physician. No action should be taken solely on the contents of this book. Always consult your physician or qualified health-care professional on any matters regarding your health and before adopting any suggestions in this book or drawing inferences from it.

The author and publisher specifically disclaim all responsibility for any liability, loss or risk, personal or otherwise, which is incurred as a consequence, directly or indirectly, from the use or application of any contents of this book.

Any and all product names referenced within this book are the trademarks of their respective owners. None of these owners have sponsored, authorized, endorsed, or approved this book.

Always read all information provided by the manufacturers' product labels before using their products. The author and publisher are not responsible for claims made by manufacturers.

Print Edition 2014

CHAPTER 1: WHAT IS SLOW COOKING?

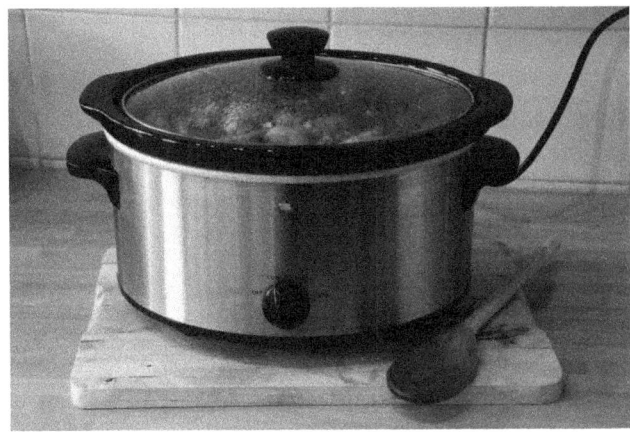

The slow cooker has been a useful appliance in the homes across the world for over 30 years. The appliance is created on the principles of cooking food slowly and the concept of it is rather simple: place the food into the pot that comes with it, and the food can be cooked slowly throughout the day. It is commonly used as a method to tenderize barbecue pit and pig roasts; the low temperatures and cooking time allows the meat to become juicy.

It is optional to be able to use a dry heat, such as that of a roaster or oven, or individuals can cook it with moisture by including a liquid into the process. The slow cooker handles the moisture in a beneficial way for the food. As it cooks, a steam is let off, and because the cooker is sealed, the collected condensation acts like a baster.

How it Works

The slow cooker originated from an electrical bean pot that was invented sometime in the 1960s with the purpose of steeping dry beans. The bean pot was created by the manufacturer, West Bend, and the style was stolen by rival company, Naxon Utilities. The bean pot was adapted to be the Crock-Pot in 1971, a slow cooker appliance that produced full meals inside of one pot. The Crock-Pot was incredibly efficient for career women who still wanted a delicious meal prepared, and this device saved them time and money. The brand rocketed into the marketing place with its capabilities; studies done by Betty Crocker Kitchen in 2002 showed that over 80% of American households were owners of at least one of these appliances.

A slow cooker is made up of three main components, these include: the outer casing, the inner container, and the lid. The outer casing is made out of metal and contains encapsulated, low-wattage heating coils. These coils have the responsibility of cooking the food. The crock is the inner container, and usually is made of glazed ceramic. This part of the cooker fits directly inside the outer heating element, and in certain models, it can be removed for easy cleaning. The last component is the domed lid, this lid fits and seals tightly onto the inner container to keep the heat from being released.

Based off of the combination of time and wattage strength, the slow cooker will cook a variety of meal options. After being turned on, heat will transfer indirectly to the electrical coils from the outer casing and lead to between the space found at the base wall and crock container. The heating will give a variable Fahrenheit degree that will be between 180 and 300. This is a conversion between 82 to 149 degrees Celsius. This is a simmering method of heating for the ingredients inside the crock. This heating for several hours at a low temperature will ensure that the food is cooked thoroughly.

While the food is cooking, steam is released, and the lid has the role of trapping it. It is an integral part of the slow cooking process by creating a vacuum seal between the rim of the crock and the lid created by the condensation. This adds extra moisture to the food and assists with the cooking process. The Crock-Pot will normally come with three settings: off, low, and high. Some slow cookers will come with programmable advancements that will automatically switch the appliance to the warm setting as soon as the food has completed cooking. This will keep the food warm until it is ready to be served, an incredibly helpful tool to have.

The Benefits

The numerous benefits of a slow cooker are astounding; such as its ability to save time while preparing nutritious and delicious meals. Individuals can place simple ingredients for a meal into the slow cooker in the morning time and have it prepared and ready to serve by the time dinner rolls around. This doesn't create much of a mess and creates less dishes to have to wash. Unlike the standard oven, the slow cooker needs only a minimal amount of electricity in order to work - therefore, using much less energy and saving money. It also doesn't heat up the whole kitchen the way and oven sometimes can and is a great safety feature against potential fires.

Another economical feature of the slow cooker is its ability to give consumers the option of purchasing more affordable cuts of meat. The condensation that is created by the cooker behaves like a self-baster and makes tougher meat become deliciously tender and far more enjoyable. Saving money and time doesn't have to mean that it's necessary to sacrifice flavor. Also, the cooker absorbs stocks and spices when cooking vegetables, giving them stronger flavors to enjoy.

Individuals can adjust the temperature with the devices low and high settings, allowing the length of cooking time to change with different meals. It is a recommendation of the U.S. Department of

Agriculture that owners cook the meal on high for the first hour, then can change the setting to low, to be sure that the food has safely and thoroughly cooked.

Slow cookers can be used for many meals, such as: meats, poultry, dips, spreads, vegetables, stews, soups, and so much more. The cooking potential with slow cookers is virtually limitless. Be sure to always thaw meats and poultry completely before cooking it in the appliance. Using a slow cooker and leaving it on all day is incredibly safe, but with all electrical devices, there are always particular dangers.

Always follow instructions for the appliance that you purchase to prevent safety hazards. This incredibly reliable cooker has made a difference in households throughout the globe. It has made it possible for women to enjoy the benefits of having a job and still providing the family with a delicious meal. Simple and easy, whether you are a professional cook or a mother, having a slow cooker is a necessity.

Chapter 2: What is the Paleo Diet?

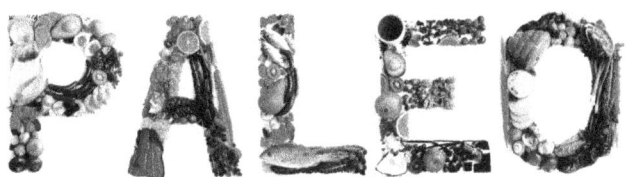

The Paleo diet, which you may have heard referred to as the caveman diet, is basically a dietary plan based on what we believe cavemen ate in the Paleolithic time period during the early half of the Stone Age.

This modern diet is composed of food groups that consist mainly of fish and other seafood, grass-fed animal meats, poultry, eggs from cage-free chickens, fruits and vegetables, nuts and seeds and healthy oils, such as flaxseed, coconut and olive oils. In a nutshell, the diet is based on the foods that could be hunted, fished and collected by cavemen thousands of years ago. Consequently, grains, legumes, dairy products, salt, refined sugar or oils, potatoes and processed foods are excluded from the diet.

Bountiful in nutrients and free from added chemicals and preservatives, research has shown that these natural food groups contribute to a healthy body. While the intention for many is losing weight on this caveman diet, the objective of living a balanced and energetic lifestyle is what keeps so many people committed. It is interesting that medical professionals recommend the same types of foods for weight control and high blood pressure today that our primitive cavemen thrived on so many years ago.

An example of a day's menu on this diet could consist of a couple of free-range eggs scrambled in olive oil with sautéed onions, peppers and mushrooms for the breakfast meal. A salad loaded with greens, veggies, nuts and sliced fruit for lunch speaks for itself in so far as the paleo diet health benefits. Dinner could be grilled salmon or other fresh fish and as many vegetables as desired seasoned with garlic and olive oil. Berries and fruits are a typical dessert or snack along with raw vegetables or nuts.

One of the first noticeable results from being on the paleo diet plan is a loss of excess fat as the body starts to convert stored fat to energy. The omissions of processed foods being replaced by all natural foods will automatically cause an upsurge in metabolism rates. People who are on the paleo diet to lose weight generally feel less hungry and do not suffer from sugar cravings. Bottom line; you are eating healthy while burning fat at the same time.

While health benefits of the paleo diet to lose weight are an incentive to undergo this strict diet, the overall health benefits are encouraging. Along with weight loss, these natural foods are recognized for their support in stabilizing blood pressure and cholesterol to healthy levels while increasing energy, a task the body cannot do when overloaded with processed foods and sugar. The distinct health benefits of this unique diet are a stronger immune defense in fighting off illness and disease, thus eliminating many health risks that are so widespread today. For whatever reason you choose for being on a diet that originated thousands of years ago, the natural foods alone will have a significant improvement on your health and vitality.

Is the diet too restrictive? It may seem that way in the very beginning, but after some time most people come to the realization that their body really doesn't need or even want these outlawed foods. It's typical for anyone to get bored by eating repetitive foods, so it's helpful to diversify your food choices as much as possible. There really is a large selection of foods on the paleo diet to choose from after all that are healthy and nutritious for your body. The diet provides the types of foods that your body needs to burn fat and feel energized which is not often found in most diets.

A paleo diet plan is not always easy to follow and probably the biggest downfall is not being able to come up with original meal ideas and staying consistent in putting together a meal plan. With the paleo diet growing in popularity there are a lot of menu plans and paleo recipe books available to help get your paleo diet journey off to a good start.

This diet is not your regular diet program that comes with a specified number of days or one you can simply get on and off anytime you wish to. Simply put this diet is more of a lifestyle choice, providing you with a solid foundation and guidelines on what you can eat and what you need to avoid. If you will take a look at the food restrictions imposed by Paleo, you will notice right away that those prohibitions actually make perfect sense, especially if you will take time to study the supporting medical reasons and explanations behind the elimination of grains, processed food, dairy and legumes from the diet.

Suffice it to say, this diet offers great benefits not just for adults, but practically for any people of any age. The diet supports the cutting down of trans-fat and hydrogenated fat, along with the reduction of glucose, carbs and hydrogenated fats.

Nevertheless, most of us also need to recognize the fact that this diet is also not any this kind of cookie cutter response or solution. Paleo food plan lays an excellent footing for you to customize meal plan depending on physical and also health and wellness considerations. As an illustration, the actual diet plan of a sportsman compared to an ordinary person can significantly vary taking into account fitness requirements and goals.

The actual eating and standard of living practices of our Paleolithic forebears provide you with a solid and sensible framework and a reference point. Changing right into a Paleo lifestyle and diet is really personal journey of sorts - of finding, understanding and adapting. Using its framework in addition to your health standards can guide you when it comes to making meals choices.

The easiest way for people not only to understand what foods are healthy and what foods are not and why, but also to grasp what it entails to be eating Paleo on a day-to-day basis. The best way to prepare a typical paleo eating plan is to map out and shop for a week's worth of meals and snacks.

Chapter 3: What are the Benefits of the Paleo Diet?

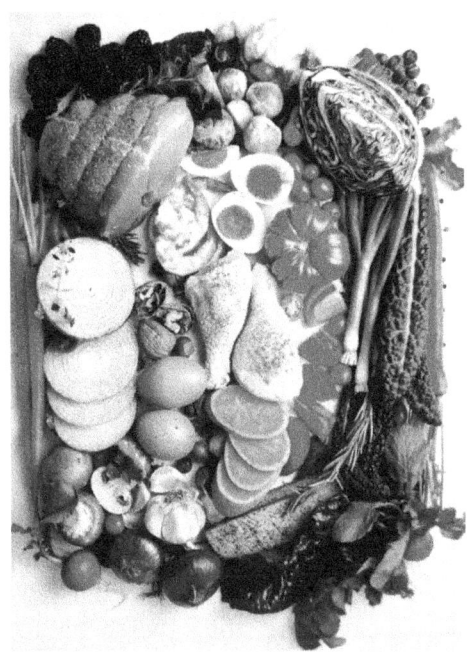

Not everyone sees the benefits of the Paleo Diet so they might not be willing to invest the time trying out the diet. This is quite unfortunate because the diet is surely one that can contribute to losing weight, getting in shape, and improving your overall health. You also eliminate the ingesting of a lot of things in modern food that really are not good for you at all.

So, Why Do Some Not See the Benefits of This Excellent Diet?

At first glance, the Paleo Diet might seem like a rather strange choice among the numerous food selections you could make. The nickname for the diet is the Caveman Diet. The notion that you would get any benefits eating the same food selections of a caveman is just too strange for most people. The reason this is so is because they have an obtuse image of what a caveman ate. They might even have very cinematic inspired images such as a caveman eating the freshly killed meat of a saber-toothed tiger. The meat is also eaten raw with the caveman eating it sitting in a cave wearing the skin of the tiger to keep warm.

This is really not what the Paleo Diet is all about. Granted, there is some truth to the image. Basically, this is a diet based on the hunter/gatherer model of acquiring food. The hunter/gatherer model of a diet is rooted in eating natural foods that do not have any processed ingredients in them. There are no refined sugars and grains are avoided. Dairy is also avoided. In the place of many common bad dietary selections, those who switch to this particular diet will be eating meat, poultry, fish, nuts, fruits, and vegetables.

In truth, many of the foods you would eat on the Paleo Diet are likely things you are already eating. You simply have to eliminate the foods that are not considered Paleo. In a way, the ease of being able to shift to a Paleo Diet from your current one might be its major benefit. On a side note, the other benefit would be you finally do get rid of a lot of truly awful food selections. Often, people eat food that is bad for them merely because they do not even know how bad it is. Once you go Paleo, a lot of the decisions are made for you. All you have to do is follow along with the diet as it is laid out.

The benefits to this diet truly are vast. Once you take time out to actually look at these many varied benefits, you just might end up being more motivated to give this unique diet a try.

The weight loss benefits to the diet are quite pronounced as long as you regulate your calorie intake and also cut back on the carbs after 4pm. There are very few carbs in this diet other than what you would find in selections of fruit. The fat content is very low except for pork and red meat selections. Overall, the food selections are low in calories. The carbs can cause weight gain, but if you taper them off later in the day, the end result is you can be more likely to lose weight.

The Paleo Diet is also a healthy one. Fish selections are loaded with omega three fatty acids. Fruits and vegetables come with a great many vitamins and nutrients. There might not be a reason to take a multivitamin if you are are eating the Paleo Diet since so many excellent vitamins and nutrients are found in the food you would commonly be eating. Of course, you do have to take steps to be sure you are eating a balanced Paleo Diet to be use you gain access to all these benefits. Eating too much of the same selections can hamper the ability to get the great benefits of the diet.

What occurs when those nutrients actually enter into the body and begin to work their magic? The truth is there are scores of different effects and many of them can improve the quality of your life. For example, your cells can be made stronger and you brain function could even improve. The better the food choices you make, the more you are going to help your body on a number of different levels. While you might not immediately see the benefits of what you are achieving through your change in diet, those benefits are taking place.

The diet is also one that is known to reduce gas and bloating. A significant number of unhealthy diet choices are notorious for their ability to cause major gas pains and problems. The best way to deal with such issues is to make the right changes to your diet. Going Paleo just might be one of the very best diet changes you could make.

There are scores of different recipes that can be made under the banner of a Paleo Diet. Even a cursory glance through a Paleo cookbook will quickly reveal there are scores upon scores of different food selections you can make. Do you wish to be very elaborate in the kitchen? You certainly have that option since there are so many unique gourmet foods you can cook up. Even holiday cooking can be done purely Paleo style.

This is not to infer that all Paleo meals are complicated to make. The truth is simply eating a banana is going Paleo. Now, you do not have to be that minimalist in your approach to eating the Paleo Diet, but it is certainly possible to make very simple, easy meals that do not require a tremendous amount of elaborate preparation.

The diet is also a very filling one. You are not likely to feel hungry since this is surely not a calorie restrictive diet with very limited food choices.

These are only a few of the major benefits that can be gained from taking part in the Paleo Diet. Why not give it a try?

Chapter 4: 10 Slow Cooker Paleo Breakfast Recipes

These are some of the best Paleo breakfast recipes you can put in your crock pot! Try one each day and please your family while keeping them fit on the Paleo diet.

BONELESS PORT SHORT RIB PALEO BREAKFAST TACOS

Ingredients:
For the Tortillas:
3 eggs, whisked
½ cup coconut milk
2 tbsp. coconut flour
Pinch of salt

For the Short Ribs:
2 pounds boneless pork short ribs
2 tbsp. maple syrup
2 tsp. garlic powder
Salt for taste

For the Toppings:
5-6 strips of bacon

1 8oz. can green chilis
2-3 tbsp. hot sauce
Chopped green onions

Directions:
Add short ribs to crock pot. Pour maple syrup, garlic powder and salt over them. Cook on low for 8-10 hours. In the morning, remove ribs from crock pot, shred and pour liquid from crock pot over shredded meat. Make the tortillas. In a medium bowl, whisk together all tortilla ingredients until smooth. Place a large skillet over medium high heat and pour ingredients into pan to create a pancake sized tortilla. Cook for approximately a minute on each side.

When tortillas are done, place bacon on the skillet and cook on both sides. Chop up cooked bacon. Mix chilies and hot sauce in a bowl, microwave for two minutes or until hot. Load up each tortilla with desired pork and toppings.

SWEET POTATO PALEO BREAKFAST CASSEROLE

Ingredients:
Coconut Oil
8 eggs
2 sweet potatoes
2 red onions
2 tbsp. smoked paprika
1 lb. meat of your choice

Directions:
Cut sweet potatoes into small pieces. Feed the onions to the food processor, and then add sweet potatoes and onions to the crock pot. Whisk eggs together and add paprika. Mix the meat into the sweet potato and onion mixture, pour the eggs in and then mix together. Cook on low heat for 4-6 hours.

PALEO APPLE SWEET POTATO SPREAD

Ingredients:
5 apples, peeled and chopped
3 sweet potatoes, peeled and chopped
¼ cup cinnamon
1 tbsp. ground ginger
1 tbsp. nutmeg
½ tsp. ground cloves

Directions:
Mix all ingredients into the crock pot and cook on low for 8 hours. Use a blender to blend recipe into a smooth spread.

PALEO FRIENDLY APPLE BUTTER

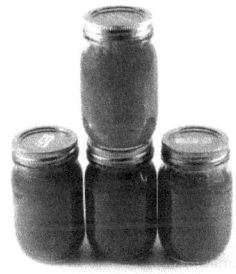

This will make a great side for any breakfast

Ingredients:
4 lbs. peeled, chopped apples
1 cup apple cider
1 tbsp. cinnamon
½ tsp. salt
¼ tsp. clove

Directions:
Place all ingredients in the crock pot. Set it to high for two hours. Turn it down to medium low for fourteen hours.

PALEO TEA EGGS

Ingredients:
12 eggs
2-4 tea bags
4 tbsp. sea salt
6 star anise
2 tbsp. cinnamon
1 tbsp. Szechuan peppercorns
1 tsp. black pepper
6-8 cups of water

Directions:
Hard boil the eggs on the stove. Cool the eggs and crack the shell but do not remove the shell. Mix tea bags, salt, cinnamon, Szechuan pepper, star anise, and black pepper in a crock pot. Add the cracked eggs; simmer on low with a lid. After 30 minutes, remove the tea bags. Cover; continue simmering for three and a half hours on low. Cool the eggs; remove shell.

EASY BREAKFAST

Ingredients:
1 sweet potato, poked
2 eggs
Pesto Ingredients:
2/3 cup walnuts
1 cup fresh basil leaves
1 peeled garlic clove
½ cup olive oil
Juice from 1/2 a lemon

Salt and pepper for taste

Directions:
Make holes in the potato with a knife or fork. Wrap potato in foil and put in the crock pot on low for 8 hours. When sweet potato is finished, remove from foil and allow it to cool. Remove the skin and mash the potato.

Make the pesto. Place walnuts, basil and garlic in a food processor and mix until leaves break apart. Slowly add olive oil. Add lemon juice, salt and pepper and mix until smooth.

Mix 2-4 tbsp. of pesto into the sweet potato. Cook an egg any style and place egg on top of sweet potato mixture.

SWEET PULLED PORK WAFFLE SLIDERS

Ingredients:
For the Pulled Pork:
2 lbs. pork butt
1 yellow onion, sliced
1 tbsp. garlic powder
1 tsp. onion powder
Salt and pepper, to taste

For the Mayonnaise:
2/3 cup avocado oil
1 egg
1 tsp. lemon juice
1 tsp. Dijon mustard
¼ tsp. garlic powder
Salt and pepper, to taste
1 tsp. maple syrup

For the Waffles:
2 cups almond flour
½ tsp. baking soda
½ tsp. garlic powder
Salt and pepper, to taste
3 eggs, whisked
½ cup canned coconut milk
2 tbsp. bacon fat
3 pieces of bacon, cooked and chopped
2 tbsp. chives, finely chopped
For the toppings:
5-6 pieces of bacon, cooked

Directions:
Place pork butt in the crock pot. Add the onions, garlic powder, onion powder, salt and pepper. Cook covered on low for 6-8 hours. Shred the pork. Make the mayonnaise and allow it to cool in the refrigerator. Place all ingredients for the mayo, except maple syrup, into tall container. Use a blender to thicken the mixture. After it thickens, add maple syrup and stir. Make waffle buns. Mix almond flour, baking soda, and garlic powder, salt and pepper together. Add eggs, coconut milk, bacon fat, chopped bacon, and chives. Mix well.

Heat up waffle iron and make waffles. Use approximately 2 tbsp. of waffle mix for each waffle. Layer waffles with ingredients and enjoy.

SPICY PALEO BREAKFAST CASSEROLE

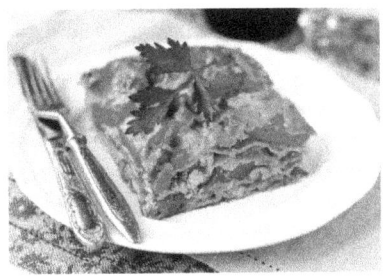

Ingredients:
1 lb. chorizo sausage
1 small onion
12 eggs
1 cup coconut milk
1 small butternut squash

Directions:
Cook the chorizo in a skillet. Add the onion when the fat of the sausage begins to sizzle. Cook until the onion is soft. The sausage will finish cooking in the crock pot. Set aside. Mix together the eggs and coconut milk. Peel, deseed and chop the squash.

Place the squash in the crock pot, then the sausage, then the egg and milk mixture. Stir it together to make sure everything is covered by the egg mixture. Turn the crock pot on low for 8-10 hours.

MAPLE BLUEBERRY BACON BREAKFAST CARNITAS

Ingredients:
2-3 lbs. pork shoulder roast
2 cups blueberries
½ cup apple juice
¼ cup maple syrup

1 tsp. cinnamon
1 tsp. dried parsley
½ tsp. dried sage
¼ tsp. nutmeg
Salt, your call
Dash of black pepper
4-5 strips of bacon
Fresh parsley, chopped

Directions:
Place pork into crock pot. Pour apple juice into pot. Add maple syrup then add cinnamon, dried parsley, dried sage, nutmeg, salt and pepper. Finish with blueberries. Cook covered on low for 8 hours. Pull out meat and shred. Use liquid from crock pot to pour over shredded meat. Cook bacon fully. Remove half the fat, saving the rest. Dice the bacon. Mix half diced bacon with the pork. Heat up remaining bacon fat. Create balls from the bacon/pork mixture and press down, creating a patty. Place in heated skillet and cook for 3-4 minutes on each side.

EASY CROCKPOT BREAKFAST PIE

Ingredients:
8 eggs, whisked
1 sweet potato or yam, shredded
1 lb. US Wellness Meats Pork Sausage, broken up
1 yellow onion, diced
1 tbsp. garlic powder
2 tsp. dried basil
Salt and pepper, to taste

Directions:
Shred the sweet potato. Add all ingredients to the crock pot and mix well. Cook covered on low for 6-8 hours.

CHAPTER 5: 10 SLOW COOKER PALEO LUNCH/DINNER RECIPES

A Paleo diet can be as rewarding and tasty as it is healthy and can easily accommodate many different forms of cooking. Slow cookers are not exempt from a Paleo enthusiast's culinary attentions. The following recipes can all be cooked in a slow-cooker, fit within the Paleo guidelines, and are absolutely scrumptious.

EASY TOMATO CHICKEN STEW

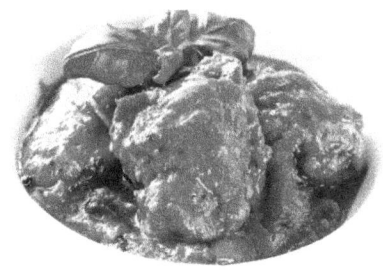

Ingredients:
1 lb. chicken thigh or breast meat
3 green bell peppers
Button mushrooms
Spicy tomato sauce, 1 tin
Salt to taste
Half a large onion

Directions:
Slice your chicken to size first. Since the slow cooker heats food so evenly you can cut the chicken as small or as big as you like without worrying about it not heating properly, though smaller cuts will cook faster. Slice your onions, bell pepper, and mushrooms. Since

the peppers and mushrooms will cook faster it is recommended you not slice them too thinly so they don't get mushy. Add all the ingredients in at once, with salt to taste. A single tin of spicy tomato sauce is usually enough; just make sure to have enough to cover the chicken. For a more watery stew simply add water, though the stew shouldn't thicken too much since water cannot escape the appliance. For 'crispy' veggies, add the vegetables in halfway through cooking.

PALEO SLOW COOKER POT ROAST

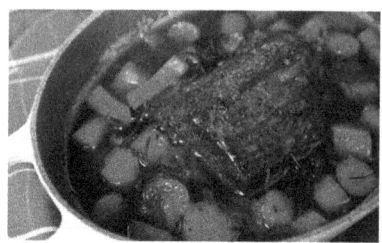

Ingredients:
1 chuck roast
6-8 medium sweet potatoes
1 large onion
1 tbsp. onion powder
1 tbsp. garlic powder
2 bay leaves
Salt (to taste)
Pepper (to taste)
2 cups orange juice
1 tbsp. ginger powder
1 tbsp. sugar
Small sprig of rosemary
1 cup baby carrots
2 and half cups water

Directions:
Slice the chuck roast into cubes. Slice the sweet potatoes and onion into cubes as well. Mix all of the dry ingredients together. Since slow cooking can blanch savory meats, thoroughly brown the meat on a stove top prior to adding it to the slow cooker. Add in the water, onion, and add in the dry ingredients. Allow the meat to cook before adding in the potatoes and carrots. This also allows you to test the broth to see if you like how it is developing. Rosemary for example, can be overpowering (depending on the (freshness of your sprig), so if you are testing the broth you can remove it before it becomes too cloying. Add the sweet potatoes and the carrots. Add orange juice midway. Cook till meat and potatoes are tender.

RED WINE STEAK STEW

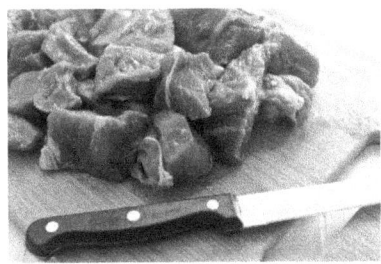

Ingredients:
1 lb. Stew beef
1 cup red wine
1 cup beef broth
1 bay leaf
1 tbsp. pepper
1 large onion
2 mashed garlic cloves

Directions:
This is a simple, hearty stew. Once you've sliced the stew into chunks, all the ingredients can be added at once and cooked till the meat is tender

THAI CHICKEN CURRY

Ingredients:
1 lb. chicken breast
2-3 medium sweet potatoes
Half a large onion
1 red bell pepper
3 tbsp. of Thai red curry paste
1 can (14oz) coconut milk

Directions:
Slice the chicken, sweet potatoes, onion and peppers. In a separate saucepan, cook the curry paste and coconut milk together. The paste is semi-solid till it melts; once the mixture is liquid in the saucepan you can transfer the sauce into the slow cooker with the other ingredients. Cook till the chicken is tender. The sweet potatoes lend themselves well to the sweet flavor of Thai curry.

MEATBALL SOUP

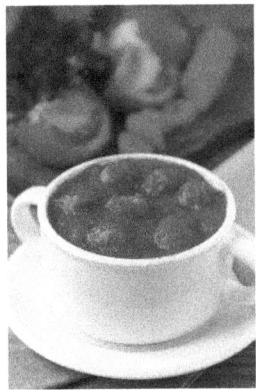

Ingredients:
1 packet ground meat
2 cups beef broth
1 can (14 oz.) tomato puree
Salt (to taste)
Pepper (to taste)
1 tbsp. cumin
1 tbsp. paprika
2 tbsp. dried oregano
3 medium tomatoes
1 large onion
4 mashed garlic gloves
2 zucchini

Directions:
Form the ground meat into uniform balls. Slice the onion thinly, chop the tomatoes roughly, and the zucchini in larger sizes. Brown the onion first, and then brown the meatballs. This way they don't stick to each other so much. Once those ingredients are browned they can all be added to the stew at once. Add the zucchini towards the end. Cook till the meatballs are cooked through and through (which will vary depending on how large you made them.

CAULIFLOWER CHICKEN SOUP

Ingredients:
3 chicken breasts
3 cups cauliflower florets
1 cup sliced carrots
Half cup celery
4 mashed garlic cloves
Salt to taste
1 cup chicken broth

Directions:
Steam the cauliflower florets first. Roughly mash the florets. Slice the chicken breasts. Add all the ingredients (minus the celery, which will be added towards the end). Cook till breasts are white through and through.

SAVORY SWEET PUMPKIN SOUP

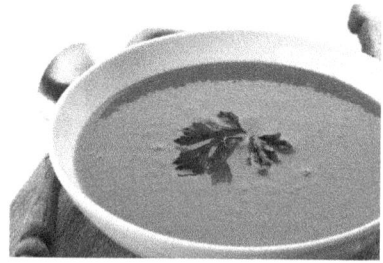

Ingredients:
2 cans (14 oz.) pumpkin puree, unsweetened
3 chicken breasts
5 sweet potatoes
1 cup sliced celery
Salt (to taste)
3 tbsp. sugar
2 cups chicken broth

Directions:
Upon slicing the chicken and the sweet potatoes all the ingredients can be added to the slow cooker at once. Add the celery towards the end since it cooks fastest.

HAM AND SPINACH STEW

Ingredients:
Half a pound pre-cooked ham
2 cups beef broth
1 cup white wine
1 cup peas
1 salad packet of spinach
Salt (to taste)
Pepper (to taste)

Directions:
Slice the ham roughly. Add all the ingredients into the slow cooker. The spinach will cook down and soften into a lovely texture. Cook till the ham is soft.

CHICKEN AND WHITE WINE STEW

Ingredients:
1 lb. chicken breasts or thigh meat
150 ml white wine
½ cup chicken broth
¼ cup Dijon mustard
Salt (to taste)
1 cup peas
1 cup carrots

Directions:
Slice all of the meat and vegetables. Add everything together at once. Cook till the chicken runs white.

SAUSAGE AND ONION SOUP

Ingredients:
2 large all beef sausages
3 onions
6 garlic cloves
2 cups beef broth
Salt (to taste)
Pepper (to taste)

Directions:
Slice the sausage. Slice the onions and brown on a stove top. Once browned you may mix the onions and all the other ingredients to the slow cooker. Cook for approximately 2 hours.

CHAPTER 6: 10 SLOW COOKER PALEO DESSERT RECIPES

There are many delightful Paleo desert recipes that can be made in a slow cooker. Below are some of the best ways one can indulge in sweets and remain on a Paleo diet.

STUFFED APPLES

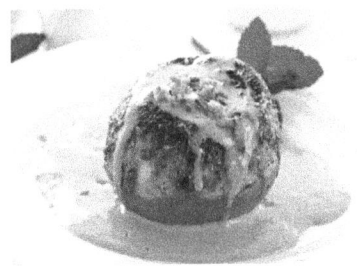

Ingredients:
Green apples, 4, cored with the bottom remaining
¼ cup of Coconut Cream Concentrated or melted coconut butter
¼ cup of unsweetened Sun butter (can substitute other nut butters)
2 tbsp. of Cinnamon
A pinch of Nutmeg
A pinch of table salt

Directions:
Core the apples with an apple corer or paring knife. Alternatively, you can cut out the top with a knife then use a spoon to scoop out the core. Do not remove the bottom of the apple. Combine the coconut butter and sun butter. Then mix in the cinnamon, nutmeg and salt. Put the cored apples in the slow cooker and add water.

Spoon the coconut and sun butter mix into the core of each apple until it reaches the top. Sprinkle cinnamon and shredded coconut over the top of the apples. Cook on low for 2 to 3 hours or until softened to desired texture.

SWIRLED CHOCOLATE ALMOND BUTTER BROWNIES

Ingredients:
¾ cup of nut almond flour
½ cup of cup cocoa powder, unsweetened
¾ tsp. of baking powder
¼ cup and an additional 2 of coconut oil, melted
½ cup of honey
1 tbsp. of vanilla
3 medium eggs
¼ cup of dark chocolate chips
3 tbsp. of nut chunky almond butter

Directions:
Place the almond flour, cocoa powder, and baking powder in a small mixing bowl. Once the dry ingredients are mixed thoroughly, pour in the vanilla. Combine the melted coconut oil and honey in another bowl and mix well. Stir in the eggs. Stir the wet and dry ingredients together, mixing thoroughly. Pour the dark chocolate chips into the mixture and stir.

Use a piece of parchment paper slightly larger than the top of the slow cooker, and press it inside. Fold it increases and cut away any that is above the edges that prevents the lid from fitting properly. Pour the brownie mixture into the slow cooker. Add the almond butter and swirl through the mixture with a knife. Cover the slow cooker and cook for an hour and a half.

PERFECTLY SLOW COOKED YAMS

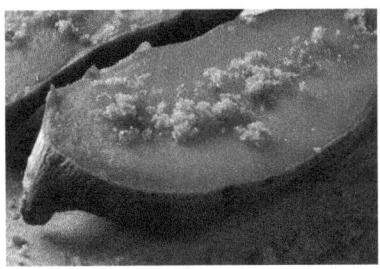

Ingredients:
Sweet potatoes or yams, 3 – 5, medium sized
Cinnamon
Almond butter or coconut butter (optional)
1 Roll of aluminum foil

Directions:
Wash and dry the yams and wrap in aluminum foil. Place the yams in the slow cooker and cook for 8 hours on low or 4 hours on high. Remove from slow cooker, slice each yam in half, lengthwise and top with almond butter and cinnamon.

SPICED APPLE SWEET POTATO

Ingredients:
5 peeled and chopped apples
3 peeled and chopped sweet potatoes
¼ cup of cinnamon
1 tbsp. of ground ginger
1 tbsp. of ground nutmeg
½ tbsp. of ground cloves

Directions:
Add all of the ingredients to slow cooker and cook on low for 8 hours. When finished cooking, pour the mixture into a blender and

mix until smooth.

BROWNIE IN A CUP

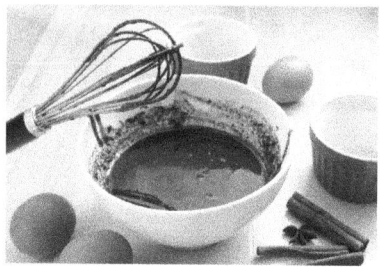

Ingredients:
½ cup of almond butter
1/8 cup of cocoa powder
1 tbsp. of vanilla extract
1 tbsp. of baking powder
A dash of salt
1 medium egg
A dash of pumpkin spice
A dash of ground ginger

Directions:
Add all of the ingredients into a mixing bowl and stir well. Use the coconut oil to grease the sides of 2 or 3 cups. Pour the batter into the cups until each is approximately half full and place them in the slow cooker. Cook on high for an hour and thirty minutes. Turn the slow cooker off and remove the lid. Let the cups cool before removing them from the slow cooker.

PALEO PUMPKIN PUDDING

Ingredients:
3 tbsp. of melted butter or coconut oil
3 cups of pumpkin, pureed

2 cups of coconut milk
3 medium eggs
½ cup of natural sweetener such as maple syrup or can substitute Stevia
2 tbsp. of pumpkin spice
1.5 tbsp. of vanilla extract
3 tbsp. of coconut flour
1 tbsp. of baking powder

Directions:
Coat the inside of the slow cooker with a small amount of the coconut oil. Place all of the ingredients in the slow cooker and stir until well mixed. For a creamier texture, you can use a blender to whip the ingredients before placing them in the slow cooker. Otherwise you can use a manual blender right in the slow cooker to blend until the lumps are removed. Cover the cooker and cook on low setting for 6 to 8 hours.

SLOW COOKED BAKED APPLES

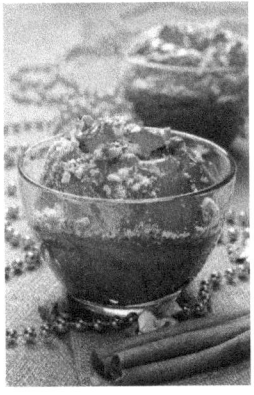

Ingredients:
6 medium apples
½ of cup raisins
1 tbsp. of cinnamon

1 tbsp. of vanilla
1 tbsp. of butter
¼ cup of almond flour
½ cup of chopped pecans
½ cup of chopped walnuts
1 tsp. of cinnamon
¼ tsp. of nutmeg
1 tbsp. of butter melted

Directions:
Core the apple then chop them into cubes. Place 1 tbsp. of butter in the slow cooker and then put in the apples, raisins, cinnamon and vanilla. Mix the ingredients. Melt the other tbsp. of butter and pour in a mixing bowl. Add the nuts, cinnamon, nutmeg and almond flour to the butter and stir using a fork. Cover the tops of the apples with the nut mixture. Cook the apples for 2 hours on high, and then reduce the setting to low and cook uncovered for another 30 minutes.

APPLE DATE CRUNCH

Ingredients:
8 small tart apples, cored and quartered
1 cup of chopped dates
1 cup of chopped pecans
1 cup of dried cherries
¼ cup of coconut oil
¼ of natural sweetener of your choice
½ cup of water
1 tbsp. of nutmeg
1 tbsp. of ground cinnamon
1 tbsp. of pumpkin spice

Directions:
Put the apples, dates, pecans and cherries into a slow cooker. Add

the nutmeg, cinnamon and pumpkin spice. Combine the coconut oil and sweetener in a sauce pan and place on low heat. Stir frequently. Add the mixture and the water to the slow cooker. Cook on high heat for 3 hours.

CHOCOLATE FLAN WITH ALMONDS

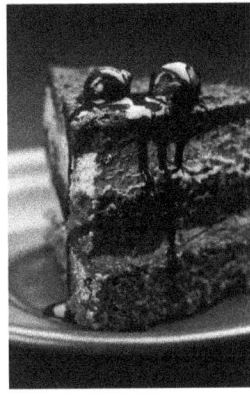

Ingredients:
2 cups of coconut sugar
1/3 cup of water
1½ cups of coconut milk
1/4 cup of toasted slivered almonds
2 eggs
2 egg yolks
3½ ounces of bittersweet chocolate

Directions for Caramel:
Pour the water and coconut sugar into a saucepan and place on medium heat. Bring to a boil. Stir until the sugar dissolves completely then let the mixture cook until it has a syrupy consistency. Pour the mixture into a dish and tilt so that all of the sides are coated with the mixture. Sprinkle the bottom of the dish with almonds.

Directions for Flan:
Put the bittersweet chocolate into an oven proof bowl. Pour the cocoa milk and sugar into a clean saucepan and bring to a boil. Stir until the sugar has dissolved. Pour the mixture on the chocolate and stir until the chocolate has melted and the mixture has a smooth consistency. Beat the eggs and egg yolks and slowly add the chocolate mixture assuring that it is mixed thoroughly with the eggs.

Pour the chocolate mixture into the dishes that have been prepared with caramel. Place aluminum foil over the tops of the dishes and set them in the slow cooker. Place the cover on the slow cooker and cook on high setting for 2 hours. Take the dishes out of the slow cooker and chill in the refrigerator overnight. To serve, loosen the flan around the edges of the dish with a knife and turn the dish upside down on a small plate to remove it.

HONEY APPLE PECAN

Ingredients:
6 medium tart apples, peeled and sliced in ½ inch pieces
1 tsp. of ground cinnamon
1/3 cup of palm sugar
½ cup of grass fed butter
½ cup of chopped pecans
½ cup of raw honey
¼ of almond flour
½ cup of shredded coconut

Directions:
Coat the inside of the slow cooker with cooking spray. Coat the apples with cinnamon and place in the slow cooker. Combine the mix coconut, flour, sugar and butter in a mixing bowl and stir with a fork until the mixture is crumbly. Mix the pecans and honey into

the mixture and spread evenly over the apples. Cook on low heat 4 to 6 hours.

APPLE CRISP

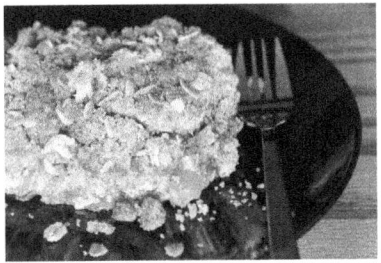

Ingredients:
4 apples, any type
¼ cup of almonds, slivered
¼ cup of almond flour
1/8 cup of coconut, shredded
3 tbsp. of cinnamon
2 tbsp. of clarified butter
Honey

Directions:
Peel the apples then core them. Next, chop them into cubes. Put the apples in a slow cooker and sprinkle cinnamon over the top of them. In a mixing bowl, combine the slivered almonds, coconut, almond flour and 2 tbsp. of cinnamon and mix thoroughly. Blend the butter into the dry ingredients and stir until the mixture becomes crumbly. Spoon the cinnamon mixture onto the apples and cook for 2 to 3 hours. Drizzle the apples with honey before serving.

ABOUT THE AUTHOR

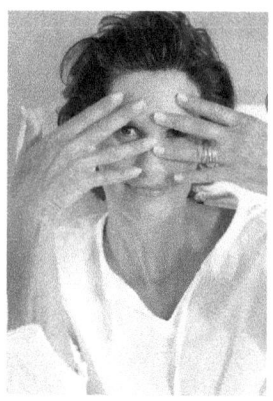

Author and chef Daisy Williams is passionate about clean and healthy eating, but she knows that it can seem next to impossible to someone just embarking on a food journey. It took years for her to move from the all-American diet processed and chemical-ridden convenience food to a healthier lifestyle that draws true nourishment from organic, whole foods. Now that she's made the transition herself, she loves helping people realize that there is a healthier way and that it's not as hard as you might think!

Eating clean didn't come easily to Daisy—her food journey started out of pure necessity. After being constantly ill for years and trying just about every medicine under the sun, she finally tried the nutrition angle as a last-ditch effort. A friend had advised reducing the chemicals in her diet, and since nothing else seemed to be working, she figured there was nothing to lose. Within weeks it became clear that nutrition was a huge factor impacting her health concerns! And thus her passion for clean eating was born.

Daisy is convinced that most people can improve their quality of life by adjusting their nutritional lifestyle. And she wants people considering clean eating to know that it's not impossible; in fact, it's delicious! Her books feature some fantastic recipes, from clean eating, green smoothies and Paleo that you'll love. Her dream is that through her story, people will be inspired to make healthy changes even before their health is suffering.

MORE BOOKS BY DAISY WILLIAMS

Clean Eating: Your Guide To Eating Clean

Clean Eating Recipes: Jumpstart Weight Loss With 70 Clean Eating Recipes

Green Smoothies: The 50 Best Green Smoothie Recipes for Weight Loss

www.ingramcontent.com/pod-product-compliance
Ingram Content Group UK Ltd.
Pitfield, Milton Keynes, MK11 3LW, UK
UKHW022120230426
12048UKWH00010BA/616